FATTY LIVER DIET FOODS LIST FOR SENIORS

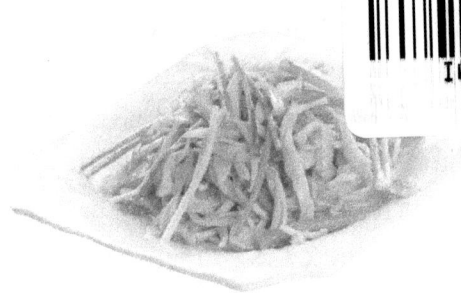

The complete pocket guide of
Delectable Recipes to Craft Your
Personalized Liver Diet and Embrace a
Liver-Friendly Lifestyle in Your Golden
Years.

Felicia O. Pace

To explore additional evidence-based and approved nutrition books similar to this one, please feel free to visit my Amazon store

https://author.amazon.com/books

TABLE OF CONTENTS

INTRODUCTION

A fatty liver diet is a crucial component in managing and mitigating the effects of fatty liver disease, a condition characterized by the accumulation of excess fat in liver cells. Whether caused by non-alcoholic factors such as obesity and metabolic syndrome or by excessive alcohol consumption, dietary choices play a pivotal role in the development and progression of this condition. A well-planned fatty liver diet focuses on promoting liver health, reducing inflammation, and supporting overall well-being.

Understanding Fatty Liver Disease

Fatty liver disease encompasses a range of conditions, from non-alcoholic fatty liver disease (NAFLD) to alcoholic fatty liver disease. NAFLD, in particular, has become increasingly prevalent due to factors such as sedentary lifestyles, poor dietary habits, and the obesity epidemic. As the liver accumulates fat, inflammation may occur, leading to more severe conditions like non-alcoholic steatohepatitis (NASH), cirrhosis, and liver failure if left unaddressed.

The Role of Diet in Fatty Liver Management

A carefully curated fatty liver diet is designed to address the root causes of liver fat accumulation and promote liver regeneration. It involves making mindful choices regarding the types of foods consumed, their nutritional content, and overall dietary patterns. The goal is to reduce fat intake, especially unhealthy fats, while prioritizing nutrient-dense foods that support liver function.

Non-Alcoholic Fatty Liver Disease (NAFLD)

Definition: NAFLD is a liver disorder that occurs in people who do not consume excessive alcohol. It ranges from simple fatty liver (steatosis) to non-alcoholic steatohepatitis (NASH), which involves inflammation and liver cell damage. If left untreated, NAFLD can progress to cirrhosis, a severe liver condition.

Causes: The primary causes of NAFLD include obesity, insulin resistance, metabolic syndrome, and elevated levels of fats in the blood (hyperlipidemia). Genetics, type 2 diabetes, and rapid weight loss are also associated risk factors.

Alcoholic Fatty Liver Disease (AFLD)

Definition: AFLD is caused by excessive alcohol consumption and is the earliest stage of alcohol-related liver disease. It can progress to more severe conditions such as alcoholic hepatitis and cirrhosis.

Causes: The main cause of AFLD is chronic alcohol abuse. The liver metabolizes alcohol, and excessive drinking can lead to the accumulation of fat in the liver cells.

Common Features of Fatty Liver Disease

Symptoms: Fatty liver disease is often asymptomatic in its early stages. As it progresses, symptoms may include fatigue, abdominal discomfort, and unexplained weight loss. In advanced stages, symptoms such as jaundice, swelling in the abdomen, and mental confusion may occur.

Diagnosis: Diagnosis typically involves a combination of medical history, physical examination, blood tests, imaging studies (ultrasound, CT scan, MRI), and sometimes a liver biopsy to assess the severity of liver damage.

Risk Factors

1. Obesity: Excess body weight, particularly abdominal obesity, is a significant risk factor for fatty liver disease.

2. Insulin Resistance: Insulin resistance, often associated with type 2 diabetes, plays a role in the development of NAFLD.

3. Metabolic Syndrome: A cluster of conditions including high blood pressure, high blood sugar, excess body fat around the waist, and abnormal cholesterol levels increases the risk.

4. Genetics: Family history can contribute to an individual's predisposition to fatty liver disease.

Prevention and Management

Healthy Lifestyle:

1. Diet: Adopting a balanced and healthy diet that includes fruits, vegetables, whole grains, and lean proteins can help manage and prevent fatty liver disease.

2. Exercise: Regular physical activity is crucial for weight management and improving insulin sensitivity.

Weight Management:
1. Losing weight, if overweight, can significantly improve liver health.
2. Gradual weight loss is recommended to prevent metabolic stress on the liver.

Controlling Medical Conditions:
- Managing conditions like diabetes, high blood pressure, and high cholesterol is important to prevent the progression of fatty liver disease.

Limiting Alcohol Intake:
- For those with AFLD, reducing or eliminating alcohol consumption is essential to prevent further liver damage.

Medications:
- Some medications may be prescribed to manage specific aspects of fatty liver disease, such as insulin sensitizers or lipid-lowering agents.

Regular Monitoring:
- Regular medical check-ups, including liver function tests and imaging studies, are crucial to monitor the progression of the disease.

APPROVED DIETARY MEAL PLANNING TIPS FOR FATTY LIVER DIET

Meal planning for a fatty liver diet involves making thoughtful choices to support liver health and reduce the risk of progression. Here are approved dietary meal planning tips for individuals with fatty liver disease:

Emphasize Whole Foods:
- Focus on whole, unprocessed foods such as fruits, vegetables, whole grains, lean proteins, and healthy fats.
- Choose a variety of colorful vegetables to ensure a range of nutrients.

Control Portion Sizes:
- Be mindful of portion sizes to avoid overeating and to maintain a healthy weight.
- Consider using smaller plates to help with portion control.

Limit Saturated and Trans Fats:
- Choose lean protein sources such as skinless poultry, fish, tofu, and legumes.
- Limit saturated fats found in red meat, full-fat dairy, and processed foods.
- Avoid trans fats found in many commercially baked and fried foods.

Incorporate Healthy Fats:
- Include sources of healthy fats such as avocados, nuts, seeds, and olive oil.
- These fats can provide essential nutrients without contributing to liver fat accumulation.

Choose Whole Grains:
- Opt for whole grains like brown rice, quinoa, oats, and whole wheat over refined grains.
- Whole grains contain fiber, which can help regulate blood sugar and improve digestion.

Moderate Sugar Intake:
- Reduce added sugars in the diet, including sugary beverages, sweets, and processed foods.
- Choose natural sweeteners like honey or maple syrup in moderation.

Monitor Carbohydrate Intake:
- Opt for complex carbohydrates found in whole grains, fruits, and vegetables.
- Control portion sizes of carbohydrates to manage blood sugar levels.

Prioritize Lean Proteins:
- Include lean protein sources such as fish, skinless poultry, tofu, beans, and legumes.
- Fish high in omega-3 fatty acids, like salmon, can be particularly beneficial.

Limit Processed Foods:
- Minimize intake of processed and packaged foods, which often contain unhealthy fats, sugars, and additives.

Increase Fiber Intake:
- Include high-fiber foods like fruits, vegetables, whole grains, and legumes to support digestion and regulate blood sugar.

Stay Hydrated:
- Drink plenty of water throughout the day to support overall health and aid in digestion.
- Limit the consumption of sugary beverages and excessive caffeine.

Balanced Meals:
- Create balanced meals that include a combination of carbohydrates, proteins, and healthy fats.
- Aim for a variety of nutrient-dense foods at each meal.

Limit Salt Intake:
- Reduce salt intake to support heart health and prevent fluid retention.
- Use herbs and spices to add flavor to meals without excessive salt.

Spread Meals Throughout the Day:
- Eat smaller, more frequent meals throughout the day to help regulate blood sugar levels.
- Avoid skipping meals to prevent overeating later.

Seek Professional Guidance:
- Consult with a registered dietitian or healthcare professional for personalized dietary advice tailored to your specific needs and condition.
- Individuals with fatty liver disease should consult with healthcare professionals to create a customized meal plan based on their health status, preferences, and dietary requirements. Regular monitoring

and adjustments to the diet may be necessary as the condition evolves

Categories of foods list to avoid or limit for fatty liver diet

When managing a fatty liver or aiming to prevent its progression, it's essential to be mindful of certain categories of foods that may contribute to liver fat accumulation or exacerbate the condition. Here's a list of food categories to generally avoid or limit in a fatty liver diet:

Highly Processed Foods:
Processed snacks, chips, and convenience foods often contain unhealthy fats, added sugars, and high levels of sodium.

Sugary Beverages:
Regular consumption of sugary drinks, including sodas, energy drinks, and certain fruit juices, can contribute to liver fat accumulation.

High-Fructose Corn Syrup (HFCS):
Foods and beverages containing HFCS, a common sweetener, should be limited as excess fructose can contribute to liver fat deposition.

Fried Foods:
Fried foods, such as French fries, fried chicken, and other deep-fried items, are high in unhealthy fats that can contribute to liver inflammation.

Fatty Meats:
Red and processed meats, particularly those high in saturated fats, can contribute to liver fat accumulation. Limit bacon, sausages, and fatty cuts of beef or pork.

High-Sugar Foods:
Foods with high sugar content, including candies, pastries, and sweetened desserts, can contribute to insulin resistance and liver fat buildup.

White Bread and Refined Grains:
Foods made with refined grains, like white bread and white rice, can spike blood sugar levels and may contribute to insulin resistance.

Full-Fat Dairy:
While dairy is an important source of nutrients, high-fat dairy products like whole milk, full-fat cheese, and cream should be consumed in moderation.

Alcohol:
Alcohol is a major contributor to liver damage, and individuals with fatty liver disease, especially alcoholic fatty liver disease, should avoid or limit alcohol consumption.

Excessive Salt:
High-sodium foods, including processed foods, canned soups, and salty snacks, can contribute to fluid retention and may exacerbate liver-related complications.

Artificial Trans Fats:
Trans fats, often found in partially hydrogenated oils, can increase levels of unhealthy cholesterol and contribute to liver inflammation. Check food labels for trans fats.

Highly Sweetened Breakfast Cereals:
Breakfast cereals with high sugar content should be avoided. Opt for whole-grain, low-sugar alternatives.

Certain Tropical Oils:
Limit the intake of oils high in saturated fats, such as palm oil and coconut oil.

Certain Fish High in Mercury:
Limit the consumption of fish high in mercury, such as shark, swordfish, king mackerel, and tilefish.

Excessive Coffee Consumption:
While moderate coffee consumption may have some benefits, excessive caffeine intake may be associated with increased liver enzyme levels in some individuals.

HEALTHY LIVER FOODS LIST

Protein

Grilled Salmon:
Protein: 25g per 3 oz
Fat: 10g
Calories: 180

Skinless Turkey Breast:
Protein: 26g per 3 oz
Fat: 1g
Calories: 135

Lean Beef (Sirloin):
Protein: 26g per 3 oz
Fat: 12g
Calories: 210

Chicken Breast (Grilled, Skinless):
Protein: 24g per 3 oz
Fat: 3g
Calories: 140

Greek Yogurt (Non-fat):
Protein: 15g per 6 oz
Fat: 0g
Calories: 80

Eggs:
Protein: 6g per large egg
Fat: 5g
Calories: 70

Tofu:
Protein: 10g per 3 oz
Fat: 5g
Calories: 94

Cottage Cheese (Low-fat):
Protein: 14g per 1/2 cup
Fat: 2g
Calories: 110

Lentils:
Protein: 18g per 1 cup (cooked)
Fat: 1g
Calories: 230

Quinoa:
Protein: 8g per 1 cup (cooked)
Fat: 4g
Calories: 222

Chickpeas:
Protein: 15g per 1 cup (cooked)
Fat: 4g
Calories: 269

Almonds:
Protein: 6g per 1 oz
Fat: 14g
Calories: 160

Walnuts:
Protein: 4g per 1 oz
Fat: 18g
Calories: 185

Flaxseeds:
Protein: 5g per 2 tbsp
Fat: 9g
Calories: 90

Soy Milk (Unsweetened):
Protein: 8g per 1 cup
Fat: 4g
Calories: 80

Vegetables

Broccoli:
Fat: 0.6g per 1 cup (cooked)
Calories: 55

Spinach:
Fat: 0.5g per 1 cup (cooked)
Calories: 41

Kale:
Fat: 0.5g per 1 cup (cooked)
Calories: 36

Brussels Sprouts:
Fat: 0.3g per 1 cup (cooked)
Calories: 56

Cauliflower:
Fat: 0.3g per 1 cup (cooked)
Calories: 27

Bell Peppers:
Fat: 0.3g per medium-sized pepper
Calories: 25

Zucchini:
Fat: 0.3g per 1 cup (cooked)
Calories: 20

Carrots:
Fat: 0.2g per 1 medium-sized carrot
Calories: 25

Cabbage:
Fat: 0.1g per 1 cup (cooked)
Calories: 22

Asparagus:
Fat: 0.2g per 1 cup (cooked)
Calories: 27

Tomatoes:
Fat: 0.4g per medium-sized tomato
Calories: 22

Cucumbers:
Fat: 0.2g per 1 cup (sliced)
Calories: 16

Sweet Potatoes:
Fat: 0.2g per 1 medium-sized sweet potato (baked)
Calories: 103

Green Beans:
Fat: 0.1g per 1 cup (cooked)
Calories: 44

Mushrooms:
Fat: 0.3g per 1 cup (sliced)
Calories: 15

Fruits

Avocado:
Fat: 14g per half avocado
Calories: 120

Berries (e.g., Blueberries, Strawberries, Raspberries):
Fat: 0.5g per cup (varies by type)
Calories: 50-80

Grapes:
Fat: 0.2g per cup
Calories: 60

Kiwi:
Fat: 0.6g per medium-sized kiwi
Calories: 50

Watermelon:
Fat: 0.2g per cup
Calories: 46

Papaya:
Fat: 0.4g per cup (cubed)
Calories: 60

Apples:
Fat: 0.2g per medium-sized apple
Calories: 95

Oranges:
Fat: 0.2g per medium-sized orange
Calories: 62

Bananas:
Fat: 0.3g per medium-sized banana
Calories: 105

Pineapple:
Fat: 0.1g per cup (chunks)
Calories: 83

Mango:
Fat: 0.6g per cup (sliced)
Calories: 107

Pears:
Fat: 0.2g per medium-sized pear
Calories: 100

Cherries:
Fat: 0.3g per cup
Calories: 87

Cantaloupe:
Fat: 0.2g per cup (cubed)
Calories: 54

Plums:
Fat: 0.2g per medium-sized plum
Calories: 30

Whole grains

Quinoa:
Fat: 3.5g per cup (cooked)
Calories: 222

Brown Rice:
Fat: 1.6g per cup (cooked)
Calories: 215

Oats:
Fat: 3.5g per cup (cooked)
Calories: 147

Barley:
Fat: 0.7g per cup (cooked)
Calories: 193

Whole Wheat Pasta:
Fat: 1.3g per cup (cooked)
Calories: 174

Bulgur:
Fat: 0.4g per cup (cooked)
Calories: 151

Farro:
Fat: 1g per cup (cooked)
Calories: 220

Millet:
Fat: 1g per cup (cooked)
Calories: 207

Amaranth:
Fat: 3.9g per cup (cooked)
Calories: 251

Whole Wheat Bread:
Fat: 1g per slice (average)
Calories: 80-100 (varies)

Buckwheat:
Fat: 1g per cup (cooked)
Calories: 155

Sorghum:
Fat: 3.4g per cup (cooked)
Calories: 143

Freekeh:
Fat: 0.7g per cup (cooked)
Calories: 130

Spelt:
Fat: 1.3g per cup (cooked)
Calories: 246

Wild Rice:
Fat: 0.6g per cup (cooked)
Calories: 166

Healthy Fat

Avocado:
Fat: 14g per half avocado
Calories: 120

Olive Oil:
Fat: 14g per tablespoon
Calories: 120

Walnuts:
Fat: 18g per 1 oz (about 14 halves)
Calories: 185

Chia Seeds:
Fat: 9g per 2 tbsp
Calories: 138

Flaxseeds:
Fat: 9g per 2 tbsp
Calories: 90

Salmon (Wild-caught):
Fat: 13g per 3 oz (cooked)
Calories: 180

Sardines (in Olive Oil):
Fat: 11g per 2 oz (canned)
Calories: 150

Almonds:
Fat: 14g per 1 oz
Calories: 160

Coconut Oil:
Fat: 14g per tablespoon
Calories: 120

Peanut Butter (Natural, Unsweetened):
Fat: 16g per 2 tbsp
Calories: 190

Dark Chocolate (70-85% Cocoa):
Fat: 12g per 1 oz
Calories: 170

Sunflower Seeds:
Fat: 14g per 1 oz
Calories: 165

Hemp Seeds:
Fat: 14g per 3 tbsp
Calories: 180

Pistachios:
Fat: 13g per 1 oz
Calories: 160

Greek Yogurt (Full-fat):
Fat: 10g per 6 oz
Calories: 150

Dairy and Dairy Alternatives

Greek Yogurt (Low-Fat or Fat-Free):

Low-Fat Greek Yogurt (6 oz): 2g fat, 100 calories

Fat-Free Greek Yogurt (6 oz): negligible fat, 80 calories

Almond Milk (Unsweetened):

Unsweetened Almond Milk (1 cup): 2.5g fat, 30 calories

Low-Fat Cheese:

Low-Fat Cheddar Cheese (1 oz): 6g fat, 50 calories

Low-Fat Mozzarella Cheese (1 oz): 4.5g fat, 50 calories

Cottage Cheese (Low-Fat):

Low-Fat Cottage Cheese (1/2 cup): 1.5g fat, 90 calories

Soy Milk (Unsweetened):

Unsweetened Soy Milk (1 cup): 4g fat, 80 calories

Skim Milk:

Skim Milk (1 cup): negligible fat, 80 calories

Low-Fat Yogurt (Flavored or Plain):

Low-Fat Fruit Yogurt (6 oz): 1.5g fat, 150 calories

Low-Fat Plain Yogurt (6 oz): 1.5g fat, 100 calories

Coconut Milk (Light):

Light Coconut Milk (1/4 cup): 3.5g fat, 50 calories

Cashew Milk (Unsweetened):

Unsweetened Cashew Milk (1 cup): 2.5g fat, 25 calories

Ricotta Cheese (Part-Skim):

Part-Skim Ricotta Cheese (1/2 cup): 10g fat, 330 calories

Probiotic Drinks:

Probiotic Kefir (Low-Fat) (1 cup): 2g fat, 110 calories

Goat Milk (Low-Fat):

Low-Fat Goat Milk (1 cup): 4g fat, 100 calories

Flax Milk (Unsweetened):

Unsweetened Flax Milk (1 cup): 2.5g fat, 25 calories

Swiss Cheese (Reduced-Fat):

Reduced-Fat Swiss Cheese (1 oz): 6g fat, 50 calories

String Cheese (Part-Skim):

Part-Skim Mozzarella String Cheese (1 piece): 6g fat, 80 calories

Beverages

Water:

Water (8 oz): negligible fat, 0 calories

Green Tea:

Unsweetened Green Tea (8 oz): negligible fat, 0 calories

Herbal Tea:

Unsweetened Herbal Tea (8 oz): negligible fat, 0 calories

Coffee:

Black Coffee (8 oz): negligible fat, 2 calories

Sparkling Water:

Sparkling Water (8 oz): negligible fat, 0 calories

Coconut Water:

Coconut Water (8 oz): negligible fat, 46 calories

Vegetable Juice:

Low-Sodium Vegetable Juice (8 oz): negligible fat, 50 calories

Tomato Juice:

Low-Sodium Tomato Juice (8 oz): negligible fat, 50 calories

Mint Infused Water:

Mint-Infused Water (8 oz): negligible fat, 0 calories

Ginger Tea:

Unsweetened Ginger Tea (8 oz): negligible fat, 0 calories

Almond Milk (Unsweetened):

Unsweetened Almond Milk (1 cup): 2.5g fat, 30 calories

Cranberry Juice (Diluted):

Diluted Cranberry Juice (8 oz): negligible fat, 50 calories

Lemon Water:

Lemon Water (8 oz): negligible fat, 0 calories

Pomegranate Juice (Diluted):

Diluted Pomegranate Juice (8 oz): negligible fat, 50 calories

Chamomile Tea:

Unsweetened Chamomile Tea (8 oz): negligible fat, 0 calories

Herbs and Spices

Basil:

Dried Basil (1 tbsp): negligible fat, 2 calories

Parsley:

Fresh Parsley (1 tbsp): negligible fat, 1 calorie

Cilantro:

Fresh Cilantro (1 tbsp): negligible fat, 0 calories

Thyme:

Dried Thyme (1 tsp): negligible fat, 3 calories

Rosemary:

Dried Rosemary (1 tsp): negligible fat, 2 calories

Oregano:

Dried Oregano (1 tsp): negligible fat, 3 calories

Turmeric:

Ground Turmeric (1 tsp): negligible fat, 9 calories

Cinnamon:

Ground Cinnamon (1 tsp): negligible fat, 6 calories

Ginger:

Fresh Ginger (1 tbsp, grated): negligible fat, 5 calories

Garlic:

Fresh Garlic (1 clove): negligible fat, 4 calories

Dill:

Dried Dill (1 tsp): negligible fat, 3 calories

Mint:

Fresh Mint (1 tbsp): negligible fat, 1 calorie

Coriander:

Ground Coriander (1 tsp): negligible fat, 5 calories

Cumin:

Ground Cumin (1 tsp): negligible fat, 8 calories

Chives:

Fresh Chives (1 tbsp): negligible fat, 1 calorie

Legumes

Lentils:

Cooked Lentils (1 cup): negligible fat, 230 calories

Chickpeas:

Cooked Chickpeas (1 cup): 4.7g fat, 269 calories

Black Beans:

Cooked Black Beans (1 cup): 0.9g fat, 227 calories

Kidney Beans:

Cooked Kidney Beans (1 cup): 0.9g fat, 225 calories

Pinto Beans:

Cooked Pinto Beans (1 cup): 1.1g fat, 245 calories

Navy Beans:

Cooked Navy Beans (1 cup): 1.0g fat, 255 calories

Cannellini Beans:

Cooked Cannellini Beans (1 cup): 0.6g fat, 220 calories

Garbanzo Beans:

Cooked Garbanzo Beans (1 cup): 2.4g fat, 269 calories

Split Peas:

Cooked Split Peas (1 cup): 0.4g fat, 231 calories

Mung Beans:

Cooked Mung Beans (1 cup): 0.4g fat, 212 calories

Adzuki Beans:

Cooked Adzuki Beans (1 cup): 0.2g fat, 294 calories

Black-eyed Peas:

Cooked Black-eyed Peas (1 cup): 0.8g fat, 160 calories

Lima Beans:

Cooked Lima Beans (1 cup): 0.4g fat, 176 calories

Great Northern Beans:

Cooked Great Northern Beans (1 cup): 0.9g fat, 209 calories

Edamame (Soybeans):

Cooked Edamame (1 cup): 8.2g fat, 189 calories

Seafoods

Salmon:

Baked or Grilled Salmon (3 oz): 6g fat, 155 calories

Mackerel:

Grilled Mackerel (3 oz): 15g fat, 305 calories

Sardines:

Canned Sardines in Water (3 oz): 11g fat, 177 calories

Trout:

Baked or Grilled Trout (3 oz): 6g fat, 144 calories

Tuna:

Canned Light Tuna in Water (3 oz): 1g fat, 73 calories

Halibut:

Baked or Grilled Halibut (3 oz): 3g fat, 77 calories

Cod:

Baked or Grilled Cod (3 oz): 1g fat, 70 calories

Shrimp:

Steamed or Grilled Shrimp (3 oz): 1g fat, 84 calories

Crab:

Steamed or Boiled Crab (3 oz): 1g fat, 85 calories

Scallops:

Baked or Grilled Scallops (3 oz): 1g fat, 95 calories

Haddock:

Baked or Grilled Haddock (3 oz): 1g fat, 74 calories

Tilapia:

Baked or Grilled Tilapia (3 oz): 2g fat, 84 calories

Clams:

Steamed or Boiled Clams (3 oz): 1g fat, 126 calories

Oysters:

Raw or Steamed Oysters (3 oz): 3g fat, 68 calories

Lobster:

Steamed or Boiled Lobster (3 oz): 1g fat, 71 calories

Sweeteners and Condiments

Sweeteners:

Honey:

1 tablespoon of Honey: negligible fat, 64 calories

Maple Syrup (Pure):

1 tablespoon of Maple Syrup: negligible fat, 52 calories

Stevia (Natural Sweetener):

1 packet of Stevia: negligible fat, negligible calories

Agave Nectar:

1 tablespoon of Agave Nectar: negligible fat, 60 calories

Date Syrup:

1 tablespoon of Date Syrup: negligible fat, 60 calories

Condiments:

Balsamic Vinegar:

1 tablespoon of Balsamic Vinegar: negligible fat, 14 calories

Mustard:

1 tablespoon of Mustard: negligible fat, 3 calories

Low-Sodium Soy Sauce:

1 tablespoon of Low-Sodium Soy Sauce: negligible fat, 10 calories

Tomato Sauce (No Added Sugar):

1/2 cup of Tomato Sauce: negligible fat, 50 calories

Salsa:

1/2 cup of Salsa: negligible fat, 20 calories

Hot Sauce:

1 tablespoon of Hot Sauce: negligible fat, 0 calories

Pesto (Light):

2 tablespoons of Light Pesto: 6g fat, 120 calories

Tahini (Unsweetened):

1 tablespoon of Unsweetened Tahini: 8g fat, 89 calories

Low-Fat Yogurt Dressing:

2 tablespoons of Low-Fat Yogurt Dressing: 2g fat, 30 calories

Guacamole:

2 tablespoons of Guacamole: 4g fat, 45 calories

Breakfast

Oatmeal with Berries and Nuts:
Oatmeal (1 cup cooked): 3.5g fat, 150 calories
Berries (1/2 cup): negligible fat, 30 calories
Nuts (1 oz): 14g fat, 160 calories

Greek Yogurt Parfait:
Greek Yogurt (6 oz): 10g fat, 150 calories
Granola (1/4 cup): 3g fat, 100 calories
Fresh Fruit (1/2 cup): negligible fat, 30 calories

Avocado Toast:
Whole Grain Bread (1 slice): 1g fat, 80 calories
Avocado (1/2 medium): 14g fat, 120 calories
Tomato slices and seasoning

Scrambled Eggs with Spinach:
Eggs (2 large): 12g fat, 140 calories
Spinach (1 cup, cooked): negligible fat, 40 calories

Whole Grain Toast (1 slice): 1g fat, 80 calories
Smoothie Bowl:
Greek Yogurt (1/2 cup): 5g fat, 80 calories
Mixed Berries (1/2 cup): negligible fat, 30 calories
Banana (1 medium): negligible fat, 105 calories

Spinach (1 cup): negligible fat, 7 calories
Almond Butter (1 tbsp): 9g fat, 90 calories

Chia Seed Pudding:
Chia Seeds (2 tbsp): 9g fat, 138 calories
Almond Milk (1 cup): 2.5g fat, 30 calories
Fresh Berries (1/2 cup): negligible fat, 30 calories

Whole Grain Pancakes with Maple Syrup:
Whole Grain Pancake (2 medium): 3g fat, 200 calories
Maple Syrup (1 tbsp): negligible fat, 52 calories
Fresh Fruit toppings

Cottage Cheese with Pineapple:
Cottage Cheese (1/2 cup): 2g fat, 110 calories
Pineapple chunks (1/2 cup): negligible fat, 40 calories

Whole Grain Cereal with Almond Milk:
Whole Grain Cereal (1 cup): 1g fat, 100 calories
Almond Milk (1 cup): 2.5g fat, 30 calories
Sliced Banana (1 medium): negligible fat, 105 calories

Quinoa Breakfast Bowl:
Quinoa (1/2 cup cooked): 3g fat, 111 calories
Almond Butter (1 tbsp): 9g fat, 90 calories
Fresh Berries (1/2 cup): negligible fat, 30 calories

Whole Grain Bagel with Smoked Salmon:
Whole Grain Bagel (1 medium): 1g fat, 200 calories
Smoked Salmon (2 oz): 3g fat, 70 calories
Cream Cheese (1 oz): 10g fat, 100 calories

Fruit and Nut Muffins:
Whole Grain Muffin (1 medium): 5g fat, 150 calories
Mixed Nuts (1 oz): 14g fat, 160 calories
Fresh Fruit (1/2 cup): negligible fat, 30 calories

Vegetable Omelette:
Eggs (2 large): 12g fat, 140 calories
Mixed Vegetables (1/2 cup): negligible fat, 30 calories
Feta Cheese (1 oz): 6g fat, 75 calories

Whole Grain Waffles with Fruit:
Whole Grain Waffle (2 medium): 3g fat, 200 calories
Mixed Berries (1/2 cup): negligible fat, 30 calories
Maple Syrup (1 tbsp): negligible fat, 52 calories

Tofu Scramble with Vegetables:
Tofu (1/2 cup, firm): 6g fat, 94 calories
Mixed Vegetables (1/2 cup): negligible fat, 30 calories
Whole Grain Toast (1 slice): 1g fat, 80 calories

Lunch

Grilled Chicken Salad:
Grilled Chicken Breast (3 oz): 3g fat, 140 calories
Mixed Greens, Tomatoes, Cucumbers
Olive Oil Dressing (1 tbsp): 14g fat, 120 calories

Quinoa and Vegetable Bowl:
Quinoa (1 cup cooked): 3g fat, 222 calories
Mixed Vegetables (e.g., broccoli, bell peppers)
Olive Oil (1 tbsp): 14g fat, 120 calories

Salmon and Asparagus:
Grilled Salmon (3 oz): 10g fat, 180 calories
Steamed Asparagus (1 cup): negligible fat, 27 calories

Turkey Wrap:
Turkey Breast Slices (3 oz): 1g fat, 90 calories
Whole Wheat Wrap
Hummus (2 tbsp): 4g fat, 50 calories
Lettuce, Tomatoes, and Cucumbers

Vegetarian Lentil Soup:
Lentils (1 cup cooked): 1g fat, 230 calories
Mixed Vegetables (carrots, celery, spinach)
Olive Oil (1 tbsp): 14g fat, 120 calories

Tuna Salad Lettuce Wraps:
Canned Tuna (3 oz): 1g fat, 100 calories
Greek Yogurt (2 tbsp): 1g fat, 20 calories
Lettuce leaves for wrapping
Chopped Celery, Red Onion

Sweet Potato and Black Bean Salad:
Roasted Sweet Potato (1 cup): 0.2g fat, 180 calories
Black Beans (1/2 cup): 0.5g fat, 110 calories
Avocado (1/4): 7g fat, 80 calories

Mediterranean Chickpea Bowl:
Chickpeas (1 cup cooked): 4g fat, 270 calories
Cherry Tomatoes, Cucumbers, Red Onion
Feta Cheese (1 oz): 6g fat, 75 calories

Veggie Stir-Fry with Tofu:
Tofu (1/2 cup): 6g fat, 94 calories
Mixed Vegetables (broccoli, bell peppers, snap peas)
Brown Rice (1/2 cup cooked): 1g fat, 108 calories

Chicken and Vegetable Skewers:
Grilled Chicken Skewers (3 oz): 3g fat, 140 calories
Zucchini, Cherry Tomatoes, Bell Peppers
Quinoa (1/2 cup cooked): 1.5g fat, 111 calories

Whole Wheat Pita with Hummus:
Whole Wheat Pita (1 medium): 1g fat, 80 calories
Hummus (3 tbsp): 9g fat, 100 calories
Sliced Cucumber and Cherry Tomatoes

Brown Rice and Vegetable Sushi Rolls:
Brown Rice (1 cup cooked): 1.6g fat, 215 calories
Nori Sheets, Avocado, Cucumber, Carrots
Soy Sauce for dipping (low sodium)

Shrimp and Quinoa Salad:
Shrimp (3 oz): 1.5g fat, 84 calories
Quinoa (1/2 cup cooked): 1.5g fat, 111 calories
Mixed Greens, Cherry Tomatoes
Lemon Vinaigrette (1 tbsp): 14g fat, 120 calories

Egg Salad Lettuce Wraps:
Hard-Boiled Eggs (2): 10g fat, 140 calories
Greek Yogurt (2 tbsp): 1g fat, 20 calories
Lettuce leaves for wrapping
Diced Celery and Red Onion

Stuffed Bell Peppers with Lean Beef:
Lean Ground Beef (3 oz): 10g fat, 210 calories
Quinoa (1/2 cup cooked): 1.5g fat, 111 calories
Bell Peppers stuffed with the mixture
Tomato Sauce (2 tbsp): negligible fat, 20 calories

Dinner

Baked Salmon with Lemon-Dill Sauce:
Salmon (4 oz): 15g fat, 240 calories
Lemon-Dill Sauce (1 tbsp): negligible fat, 10 calories
Steamed Broccoli (1 cup): negligible fat, 55 calories

Vegetable Stir-Fry with Tofu:
Tofu (1 cup): 12g fat, 190 calories
Mixed Vegetables (broccoli, bell peppers, snap peas)
Brown Rice (1 cup cooked): 1.5g fat, 215 calories

Grilled Chicken Breast with Quinoa Salad:
Grilled Chicken Breast (4 oz): 6g fat, 180 calories
Quinoa Salad with Vegetables
Olive Oil (1 tbsp for dressing): 14g fat, 120 calories

Turkey and Vegetable Skillet:
Ground Turkey (4 oz): 16g fat, 280 calories
Mixed Vegetables (zucchini, bell peppers, carrots)
Quinoa (1/2 cup cooked): 1.5g fat, 111 calories

Mushroom and Spinach Stuffed Chicken Breast:
Chicken Breast (6 oz): 4g fat, 220 calories
Mushroom and Spinach Stuffing
Baked Sweet Potato (1 medium): 0.2g fat, 103 calories

Lentil and Vegetable Curry:
Lentils (1 cup cooked): 1g fat, 230 calories
Mixed Vegetables (cauliflower, peas, carrots)
Brown Rice (1/2 cup cooked): 1.5g fat, 108 calories

Chickpea and Spinach Salad:
Chickpeas (1 cup cooked): 4g fat, 270 calories
Fresh Spinach, Cherry Tomatoes, Cucumber
Feta Cheese (1 oz): 6g fat, 75 calories

Salmon and Quinoa Stuffed Bell Peppers:
Canned Salmon (5 oz): 15g fat, 345 calories
Quinoa (1/2 cup cooked): 1.5g fat, 111 calories
Bell Peppers stuffed with the mixture

Eggplant and Tomato Bake:
Eggplant Slices (1 medium): negligible fat, 20 calories
Tomato Slices, Basil, Mozzarella Cheese (1 oz): 6g fat, 85 calories
Olive Oil Drizzle (1 tbsp): 14g fat, 120 calories

Shrimp and Broccoli Stir-Fry:
Shrimp (4 oz): 1g fat, 100 calories
Broccoli, Snap Peas, Carrots
Brown Rice (1/2 cup cooked): 1.5g fat, 108 calories

Grilled Vegetable and Quinoa Bowl:
Mixed Grilled Vegetables (zucchini, bell peppers, eggplant)
Quinoa (1 cup cooked): 3g fat, 222 calories
Hummus (2 tbsp): 4g fat, 50 calories

Pesto Pasta with Cherry Tomatoes:
Whole Wheat Pasta (1 cup cooked): 2g fat, 174 calories
Pesto Sauce (2 tbsp): 18g fat, 150 calories
Cherry Tomatoes, Pine Nuts (1 oz): 14g fat, 160 calories

Cauliflower Rice Stir-Fry with Chicken:
Chicken Breast (4 oz): 6g fat, 180 calories
Cauliflower Rice (1 cup cooked): 2g fat, 28 calories
Mixed Vegetables (bell peppers, peas, carrots)

Lemon Herb Baked Cod:
Cod Fillet (4 oz): 0.5g fat, 100 calories
Lemon-Herb Marinade
Steamed Asparagus (1 cup): negligible fat, 27 calories

Bean and Vegetable Chili:
Mixed Beans (black beans, kidney beans, pinto beans - 1 cup): 1g fat, 218 calories
Tomatoes, Onions, Bell Peppers
Avocado (1/4): 7g fat, 80 calories

Snacks and Appetizer

Guacamole with Veggie Sticks:
Avocado (1 medium): 14g fat, 240 calories
Carrot and Celery Sticks for dipping

Hummus and Whole Wheat Pita:
Hummus (2 tbsp): 4g fat, 50 calories
Whole Wheat Pita (1 small): 1g fat, 80 calories

Greek Yogurt with Berries:
Greek Yogurt (6 oz): 10g fat, 150 calories
Mixed Berries (1/2 cup): negligible fat, 30 calories

Cucumber Slices with Tzatziki:
Tzatziki Sauce (2 tbsp): 6g fat, 60 calories
Cucumber slices for dipping

Almonds and Dried Fruit Mix:
Almonds (1 oz): 14g fat, 160 calories
Dried Apricots and Cranberries (1/4 cup): negligible fat, 60 calories

Baked Sweet Potato Fries:
Sweet Potato (1 medium): 0.2g fat, 103 calories
Olive Oil (1 tbsp for baking): 14g fat, 120 calories

Caprese Skewers:
Cherry Tomatoes, Mozzarella Cheese (1 oz): 6g fat, 85 calories
Basil leaves, Balsamic Glaze drizzle

Hard-Boiled Eggs:
Hard-Boiled Eggs (2): 10g fat, 140 calories

Whole Grain Crackers with Cheese:
Whole Grain Crackers (1 oz): 5g fat, 110 calories
Cheese (1 oz): 9g fat, 110 calories

Celery with Peanut Butter:
Celery Sticks: negligible fat, 10 calories
Peanut Butter (2 tbsp): 16g fat, 180 calories

Sliced Apple with Almond Butter:
Apple Slices (1 medium): negligible fat, 95 calories
Almond Butter (1 tbsp): 9g fat, 90 calories

Tomato Bruschetta on Whole Wheat Toast:
Tomatoes, Basil, Garlic, Olive Oil (1 tbsp): 14g fat, 120 calories
Whole Wheat Baguette Slice

Mixed Nuts:
Mixed Nuts (1 oz): 14g fat, 160 calories

Vegetable Spring Rolls with Dipping Sauce:
Rice Paper Wrappers, Shredded Veggies (cabbage, carrots, bell peppers)
Dipping Sauce (low sodium soy sauce with a dash of sesame oil)

Smoked Salmon Rolls:
Smoked Salmon (2 oz): 3g fat, 70 calories
Cream Cheese (1 oz): 10g fat, 100 calories
Cucumber Slices for rolling

Soup and stew

Vegetable Lentil Soup:
Lentils (1 cup cooked): 1g fat, 230 calories
Mixed Vegetables (carrots, celery, tomatoes)
Vegetable Broth

Minestrone Soup:
Whole Wheat Pasta (1/2 cup cooked): 1g fat, 100 calories
Kidney Beans, Tomatoes, Spinach
Vegetable Broth

Chicken and Vegetable Soup:
Chicken Breast (3 oz): 3g fat, 140 calories
Mixed Vegetables (carrots, celery, peas)

Chicken Broth

Sweet Potato and Black Bean Stew:
Sweet Potatoes (1 cup): 0.2g fat, 180 calories
Black Beans (1/2 cup cooked): 0.5g fat, 110 calories
Tomatoes, Onion, Vegetable Broth

Tomato Basil Soup:
Tomatoes, Basil, Garlic, Onion
Olive Oil (1 tbsp): 14g fat, 120 calories
Vegetable Broth

Salmon Chowder:
Salmon (3 oz): 10g fat, 180 calories
Potatoes, Corn, Celery
Low-Fat Milk

Curried Cauliflower Soup:
Cauliflower (1 cup): 0.3g fat, 27 calories
Coconut Milk (1/4 cup): 6g fat, 60 calories
Curry Spices

Mushroom Barley Soup:
Barley (1/2 cup cooked): 0.5g fat, 97 calories
Mushrooms, Carrots, Celery
Vegetable Broth

Turkey Chili:
Ground Turkey (4 oz): 16g fat, 280 calories
Kidney Beans, Tomatoes, Chili Spices

Low-Sodium Chicken Broth

Quinoa and Vegetable Stew:
Quinoa (1/2 cup cooked): 3g fat, 111 calories
Mixed Vegetables (zucchini, bell peppers, carrots)
Vegetable Broth

Chicken and Brown Rice Congee:
Chicken Thighs (3 oz): 6g fat, 140 calories
Brown Rice (1/2 cup cooked): 1.5g fat, 108 calories
Ginger, Garlic, Chicken Broth

Black-Eyed Pea Soup:
Black-Eyed Peas (1 cup cooked): 1g fat, 194 calories
Collard Greens, Tomatoes
Vegetable Broth

Butternut Squash Soup:
Butternut Squash (1 cup): 0.2g fat, 63 calories
Carrots, Onion, Ginger
Vegetable Broth

Shrimp and Vegetable Gumbo:
Shrimp (4 oz): 1g fat, 100 calories
Okra, Bell Peppers, Tomatoes
Cajun Spices, Chicken Broth

Bean and Kale Soup:
Cannellini Beans (1 cup cooked): 0.6g fat, 218 calories
Kale, Tomatoes, Onion
Vegetable Broth

Desserts

Baked Apples with Cinnamon:
Apples (1 medium): negligible fat, 95 calories
Cinnamon and a touch of honey

Greek Yogurt Parfait:
Greek Yogurt (6 oz): 10g fat, 150 calories
Fresh Berries (1/2 cup): negligible fat, 30 calories
Granola (1/4 cup): 3g fat, 100 calories

Chia Seed Pudding with Berries:
Chia Seeds (2 tbsp): 9g fat, 138 calories
Almond Milk (1 cup): 2.5g fat, 30 calories
Mixed Berries (1/2 cup): negligible fat, 30 calories

Banana Oat Cookies:
Mashed Banana (1 medium): negligible fat, 105 calories
Rolled Oats (1/2 cup): 3g fat, 154 calories
Cinnamon, Vanilla Extract

Dark Chocolate-Dipped Strawberries:
Strawberries (1 cup): negligible fat, 50 calories
Dark Chocolate (1 oz, 70-85% cocoa): 12g fat, 170 calories

Pumpkin Custard:
Canned Pumpkin (1/2 cup): 0.5g fat, 40 calories
Eggs (2): 10g fat, 140 calories
Cinnamon, Nutmeg, and a touch of honey

Coconut and Mango Sorbet:
Mango (1 cup, frozen): negligible fat, 100 calories
Coconut Milk (1/4 cup): 13g fat, 120 calories

Mixed Berry Smoothie Bowl:
Mixed Berries (1/2 cup): negligible fat, 30 calories
Greek Yogurt (1/2 cup): 5g fat, 80 calories
Granola (1/4 cup): 3g fat, 100 calories

Almond Flour Blueberry Muffins:
Almond Flour (1 cup): 80g fat, 640 calories
Blueberries (1/2 cup): negligible fat, 40 calories
Eggs (2) and a touch of honey

Avocado Chocolate Mousse:
Avocado (1 medium): 14g fat, 240 calories
Cocoa Powder (2 tbsp): 1.5g fat, 20 calories
Maple Syrup (1 tbsp): negligible fat, 52 calories

Raspberry Oat Bars:
Rolled Oats (1 cup): 6g fat, 300 calories
Raspberry Jam (1/2 cup, no added sugar):
negligible fat, 120 calories

Frozen Yogurt Bites:
Greek Yogurt (1 cup): 10g fat, 150 calories
Mixed Berries (1/2 cup): negligible fat, 30
calories

Cinnamon Baked Pears:
Pears (1 medium): negligible fat, 100 calories
Cinnamon, a touch of honey

Walnut and Date Energy Balls:
Walnuts (1/2 cup): 33g fat, 383 calories
Dates (1/2 cup, pitted): negligible fat, 200
calories

Lemon Sorbet:
Lemon Juice (1/2 cup): negligible fat, 8 calories
Simple Syrup (1/4 cup): negligible fat, 50
calories

BONUS: SHOPPING LIST

Creating a shopping list for a fatty liver diet involves selecting nutrient-dense, whole foods while minimizing processed and high-fat items. Here's a diverse shopping list that includes a variety of foods suitable for a fatty liver diet:

Fresh Produce:

1. Spinach
2. Kale
3. Broccoli
4. Brussels Sprouts
5. Avocado
6. Berries (blueberries, strawberries)
7. Apples
8. Oranges

Vegetables:

1. Bell Peppers
2. Zucchini
3. Carrots
4. Cauliflower
5. Sweet Potatoes
6. Tomatoes

7. Cucumbers

Whole Grains:

1. Quinoa
2. Brown Rice
3. Oats
4. Barley
5. Whole Wheat Bread
6. Bulgur

Lean Proteins:

1. Skinless Chicken Breast
2. Turkey
3. Fish (salmon, trout)
4. Tofu
5. Lentils
6. Chickpeas
7. Eggs

Dairy and Alternatives:

1. Greek Yogurt (low-fat or fat-free)
2. Almond Milk (unsweetened)
3. Low-Fat Cheese
4. Cottage Cheese

Healthy Fats:

1. Olive Oil
2. Avocado Oil
3. Nuts (almonds, walnuts)
4. Seeds (flaxseeds, chia seeds)

Fruits:

1. Bananas
2. Mangoes
3. Grapes
4. Kiwi
5. Pears

Herbs and Spices:

1. Garlic
2. Ginger
3. Turmeric
4. Cinnamon
5. Basil
6. Parsley

Legumes:

1. Black Beans
2. Kidney Beans
3. Chickpeas
4. Lentils

Seafood:

1. Shrimp
2. Cod
3. Sardines

Whole Wheat Pasta:

1. Whole Wheat Spaghetti
2. Brown Rice Noodles

Condiments:

1. Balsamic Vinegar
2. Mustard
3. Low-Sodium Soy Sauce
4. Tomato Sauce (no added sugar)

Beverages:

1. Green Tea
2. Herbal Tea
3. Water

Snacks:

1. Almond Butter
2. Hummus
3. Rice Cakes
4. Greek Yogurt Parfait Ingredients (see previous list)

Sweeteners:

1. Honey
2. Maple Syrup (in moderation)

Deli:

1. Lean Deli Meats (turkey, chicken)
2. Whole Grain Wraps

Canned Goods:

1. Low-Sodium Vegetable Broth
2. Canned Tuna (in water)

Frozen Foods:

1. Frozen Berries
2. Frozen Vegetables (mixed varieties)
3. Frozen Fish Fillets

Grass-Fed Meat:

1. Grass-Fed Beef
2. Grass-Fed Lamb

Dried Fruits:

1. Dried Apricots (unsweetened)
2. Raisins (in moderation)

CONCLUSION

In conclusion, adopting a fatty liver diet tailored for seniors is a proactive and empowering approach to support liver health and overall well-being. By embracing a diet rich in nutrient-dense foods, practicing portion control, and making mindful food choices, seniors can play a pivotal role in managing fatty liver disease and mitigating associated risks. This dietary journey involves a commitment to whole, unprocessed foods, moderation in sugar and unhealthy fats, and a balanced distribution of macronutrients.

As we age, prioritizing liver health becomes increasingly vital, and a well-thought-out diet is a valuable tool in maintaining optimal liver function. Seniors are encouraged to collaborate with healthcare professionals or registered dietitians to create personalized dietary plans that align with their unique needs, medical conditions, and lifestyle.

By adopting a liver-friendly diet, seniors not only take charge of their liver health but also contribute to enhanced overall health, energy levels, and vitality. Regular monitoring, combined with a commitment to making informed food choices, forms the foundation for a healthier, more vibrant life in the senior years.

Remember, the journey toward better liver health is a holistic one, and a well-balanced diet is a key ally in this pursuit.

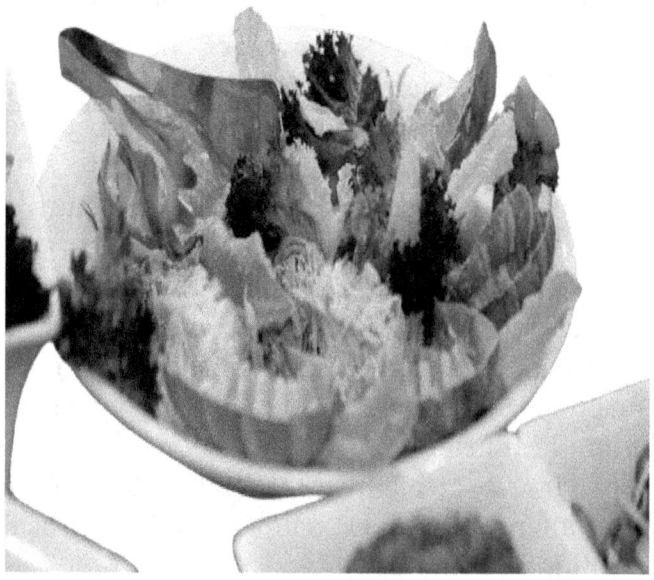

Dear Cherished Readers

I trust this book has served as a wellspring of inspiration, solace, and valuable insights for you. Each recipe was crafted with love, meticulous attention to detail, and a profound understanding of effective utilization ensuring wholesome and nutritious meals.

Your reviews, experiences, and insights are invaluable. Every evaluation propels me to enhance and tailor my work to better cater to your needs. Let's engage in a meaningful discussion—a dialogue that transcends the written words, forging a deeper connection. Your thoughts are the driving force behind continuous improvement.

Warm regards,

Felicia O. Pace

To explore additional evidence-based and approved nutrition books similar to this one, please feel free to visit my Amazon store

https://author.amazon.com/books